Table of Contents

Mastery of the basic understanding of carbohydrate counting includes understanding the relationship among food, physical activity, and blood glucose levels. Advanced carbohydrate counting includes understanding pattern management and how to use insulin-to-carbohydrate ratios.

Basic carbohydrate counting helps patients get started with the carbohydrate counting system. Carbohydrate foods are identified as starches, fruit, milk, and desserts. Emphasis is placed on consistency in the timing, type, and amount of carbohydrate-containing foods consumed. Early on, discussion of portion sizes is also key to understanding the concept of what a serving of carbohydrate is. Carbohydrates are measured in grams and may be referred to in grams or servings. One carbohydrate serving is equal to 15 g of carbohydrate.

Counting calories might be something you've already done at one time or another in your life. Counting carbohydrates may be something new to you. So why is counting carbohydrates so important when you have diabetes?

Understanding Blood Glucose Level

Diabetes

Diabetes is defined as a disease in which the body has an impaired ability to either produce or respond to the hormone insulin. People with type 1 diabetes have a pancreas that does not make insulin. People with type 2 diabetes have cells in the body that are resistant to insulin or have a pancreas that slows or stops producing adequate insulin levels (blood glucose).

Both types of diabetes can result in abnormal glucose levels.

Normal blood levels may range slightly depending on what blood tests are used, and your doctor may have, but the variances are small. In addition, what are "normal" ranges for nondiabetics are not the same for diabetics; it is generally accepted that target blood sugar measurements for people with diabetes will be slightly higher than those without diabetes.

A person who is does not have a normal glucose range of 72-99 mg/dL while fasting and up to 140 mg/dL about 2 hours after eating. People with diabetes who have well-controlled glucose levels with medications have a different target glucose range. These people may have a fasting range of about 100 mg/dL or less and 180 mg/dL about 2 hours after eating. If a person's diabetes is not well controlled, the person may have much higher glucose ranges or hypoglycemia (for example, 200 -400 mg/d; however some people with diabetes have blood sugar levels that are much higher.

Diagnosis

Symptoms of type 1 diabetes often appear suddenly and are often the reason for checking blood sugar levels. Because symptoms of other types of diabetes and prediabetes come on more gradually or may not be evident, the American Diabetes Association (ADA) has recommended screening guidelines. The ADA recommends that the following people be screened for diabetes:

Anyone with a body mass index higher than 25 (23 for Asian Americans), regardless of age, who has additional risk factors, such as high blood pressure, abnormal cholesterol levels, a sedentary lifestyle, a history of polycystic ovary syndrome or heart disease, and who has a close relative with diabetes.

Anyone older than age 45 is advised to receive an initial blood sugar screening, and then, if the results are normal, to be screened every three years thereafter.

Women who have had gestational diabetes are advised to be screened for diabetes every three years.

Anyone who has been diagnosed with prediabetes is advised to be tested ever.

Understanding blood glucose level ranges can be a key part of diabetes self-management.

Tests for type 1 and type 2 diabetes and prediabetes

Glycated hemoglobin (A1C) test. This blood test, which doesn't require fasting, indicates your average blood sugar level for the past two to three months. It measures the percentage of blood sugar attached to hemoglobin, the oxygen-carrying protein in red blood cells.

The higher your blood sugar levels, the more hemoglobin you'll have with sugar attached. An A1C level of 6.5% or higher on two separate tests indicates that you have diabetes. An A1C between 5.7 and 6.4 % indicates prediabetes. Below 5.7 is considered normal.

If the A1C test results aren't consistent, the test isn't available, or you have certain conditions that can make the A1C test inaccurate — such as if you are pregnant or have an uncommon form of hemoglobin (known as a hemoglobin variant) — your doctor may use the following tests to diagnose diabetes:

Random blood sugar test.

A blood sample will be taken at a random time. Regardless of when you last ate, a blood sugar level of 200 milligrams per deciliter (mg/dL) — 11.1 millimoles per liter (mmol/L) — or higher suggests diabetes.

Fasting blood sugar test.

A blood sample will be taken after an overnight fast. A fasting blood sugar level less than 100 mg/dL (5.6 mmol/L) is normal. A fasting blood sugar level from 100 to 125 mg/dL (5.6 to 6.9 mmol/L) is considered prediabetes. If it's 126 mg/dL (7 mmol/L) or higher on two separate tests, you have diabetes.

Oral glucose tolerance test.

For this test, you fast overnight, and the fasting blood sugar level is measured. Then you drink a sugary liquid, and blood sugar levels are tested periodically for the next two hours.

A blood sugar level less than 140 mg/dL (7.8 mmol/L) is normal. A reading of more than 200 mg/dL (11.1 mmol/L) after two hours indicates diabetes. A reading between 140 and 199 mg/dL (7.8 mmol/L and 11.0 mmol/L) indicates prediabetes.

If type 1 diabetes is suspected, your urine will be tested to look for the presence of a byproduct produced when muscle and fat tissue are used for energy because the body doesn't have enough insulin to use the available glucose (ketones). Your doctor will also likely run a test to see if you have the destructive immune system cells associated with type 1 diabetes called autoantibodies.

Tests for gestational diabetes

Your doctor will likely evaluate your risk factors for gestational diabetes early in your pregnancy:

If you're at high risk of gestational diabetes — for example, if you were obese at the start of your pregnancy; you had gestational diabetes during a previous pregnancy; or you have a mother, father, sibling or child with diabetes — your doctor may test for diabetes at your first prenatal visit.

If you're at average risk of gestational diabetes, you'll likely have a screening test for gestational diabetes sometime during your second trimester — typically between 24 and 28 weeks of pregnancy.

Your doctor may use the following screening tests:

Initial glucose challenge test. You'll begin the glucose challenge test by drinking a syrupy glucose solution. One hour later, you'll have a blood test to measure your blood sugar level. A blood sugar level below 140 mg/dL (7.8 mmol/L) is usually considered normal on a glucose challenge test, although this may vary at specific clinics or labs.

If your blood sugar level is higher than normal, it only means you have a higher risk of gestational diabetes. Your doctor will order a follow-up test to determine if you have gestational diabetes.

Follow-up glucose tolerance testing. For the follow-up test, you'll be asked to fast overnight and then have your fasting blood sugar level measured. Then you'll drink another sweet solution — this one containing a higher concentration of glucose — and your blood sugar level will be checked every hour for a period of three hours.

If at least two of the blood sugar readings are higher than the normal values established for each of the three hours of the test, you'll be diagnosed with gestational diabetes.

Recommended target blood glucose level ranges

The NICE recommended target blood glucose levels are stated below for adults with type 1 diabetes, type 2 diabetes and children with type 1 diabetes.

In addition, the International Diabetes Federation's target ranges for people without diabetes is stated.

Normal and diabetic blood sugar ranges

For the majority of healthy individuals, normal blood sugar levels are as follows:

Between 4.0 to 5.4 mmol/L (72 to 99 mg/dL) when fasting [361]

Up to 7.8 mmol/L (140 mg/dL) 2 hours after eating

For people with diabetes, blood sugar level targets are as follows:

Before meals : 4 to 7 mmol/L for people with type 1 or type 2 diabetes

After meals : under 9 mmol/L for people with type 1 diabetes and under 8.5mmol/L for people with type 2 diabetes.

How does food affect blood sugar levels?

Many factors, including exercise, stress, and illness, affect your blood sugar levels.

That said, one of the largest factors is what you eat.

Of the three macronutrients — carbs, protein, and fat — carbs have the greatest effect on blood sugar. That's because your body breaks down carbs into sugar, which enters your bloodstream.

This occurs with all carbs, such as refined sources like chips and cookies, as well as healthy types like fruits and vegetables.

However, whole foods contain fiber. Unlike starch and sugar, naturally occurring fiber does not raise blood sugar levels and may even slow this rise.

When people with diabetes eat foods high in digestible carbs, their blood sugar levels can surge. High carb intake typically requires high doses of insulin or diabetes medication to control blood sugar.

Given that they're unable to produce insulin, people with type 1 diabetes need to inject insulin several times a day, regardless of what they eat. However, eating fewer carbs can significantly reduce their mealtime insulin dosage.

Carbohydrate counting is a way to keep track of the carbohydrates in food and gain control of blood sugar. With some practice, the amount of insulin needed can be determined by figuring out the amount of carbohydrates in a meal.

Counting carbs

- Keeps you in control of your blood sugar
- Keeps you in balance with with your medication or insulin dose
- Keeps you in control of food portions to manage your body weigh

who is a candidate for carbohydrate counting?

Anyone using Humalog/rapid actin insulin, which is injected at the time of eating. This may vary with each individual.

Anyone using an insulin pump.

Anyone whose blood sugar levels are not within normal range with current eating patterns.

If you take mealtime insulin, you'll count carbs to match your insulin dose to the amount of carbs in your foods and drinks. You may also take additional insulin if your blood sugar is higher than your target when eating.

What are the different types of carbs

There are 3 types of carbs:

Sugars, such as the natural sugar in fruit and milk or the added sugar in soda and many other packaged foods.

Starches, including wheat, oats, and other grains; starchy vegetables such as corn and potatoes; and dried beans, lentils, and peas.

Fiber, the part of plant foods that isn't digested but helps you stay healthy.

Sugars and starches raise your blood sugar, but fiber doesn't.

What are carbohydrates

Carbohydrate is sugar – and includes both single sugar units called sugar (or glucose) and chains of sugar units chemically linked together called starch. Carbohydrate has to be broken down into single sugar units to be absorbed. Glucose is the most common sugar unit in our food and in our bodies.

Every carbohydrate we eat is converted into glucose and has an impact on blood sugar levels.

Carbohydrates are commonly found within the following foods:

Rice

grains

cereals and pasta

Breads, tortillas, crackers, bagels and rolls

Dried beans, split peas and lentils

Vegetables, like potatoes, corn, peas and winter squash

Fruit

Milk

Yogurt

Sugars, like table sugar and honey

Foods and drinks made with sugar, like regular soft drinks and desserts

Fiber

What about fiber? Fiber is a complex carbohydrate found in fruit, vegetables and whole grains. However, while you can eat fiber, you do not digest it. It will not cause your blood sugar levels to rise, so you do not need to take insulin to cover the fiber.

HOW IS CARBOHYDRATE COUNTING DONE?

Carbs are measured in grams. On packaged foods, you can find total carb grams on the Nutrition Facts label. You can also check this list or use a carb-counting app to find grams of carbs in foods and drinks.

For diabetes meal planning, 1 carb serving is about 15 grams of carbs. This isn't always the same as what you think of as a serving of food. For example, most people would count a small baked potato as 1 serving. However, at about 30 grams of carbs, it counts as 2 carb servings.

Know which foods contain carbohydrates.

Starches (breads, cereals, grains, legumes, and starchy vegetables like corn and peas)

Fruits and juices

Milk and yogurt

Pies, cakes, candy, ice cream, etc.

Know portion sizes. Use a carbohydrate counter and measure your food. One serving of carbohydrates = 15 grams. The following are equivalent to one carbohydrate serving:

1/2 cup of starch (e.g. potatoes, corn, peas, grains)

1 slice of bread

1 small piece of fruit

8 oz. milk or yogurt

1 1/2 cups of cooked vegetables

Estimate a reasonable carbohydrate intake per meal depending on height, weight, gender, age, and activity level.

An average female needs 45—60 grams of carbohydrate per meal, or more with increased activity (in the form of a snack or a slightly larger meal).

An average male needs 60—80 grams of carbohydrate per meal, or more with increased activity.

A diabetes management team will be able to help determine this more precisely.

Check blood sugar levels 1—2 hours after eating, particularly after eating too many carbohydrates. This is the peak time for carbohydrate digestion.

Eat balanced meals that include more whole foods and less processed foods.

Eat healthy fats. With much recent research showing the advantage of lower carbohydrate diets, consider adding more healthy fats and protein to prevent elevated blood sugar levels.

Remember that sugar-free does not mean carbohydrate free. The total number of carbohydrates eaten will impact blood sugar levels, no matter whether they come from sugars, starches, or fruits.

Basic carb counting

Basic carb counting can help you learn how certain foods affect your blood glucose levels, and the aim is to eat a consistent amount of carbs each day. This is most likely to be adopted by people with non-insulin treated type 2 diabetes.

A dietitian can advise you on how much carbohydrate you should eat at each meal based on your medication, weight goals and overall diabetes control. In the interim, you could ask your doctor for an appropriate amount of carbs (e.g. 45-60 grams per day) to eat at each meal before your meeting with a dietitian.

Consistent carb counting

Consistent carb counting, also known as advanced carb counting, can be used by people with diabetes who are treated with rapid-acting insulin. To count carbs, you will use an insulin-to-carb ratio, which calculates how much insulin you need to cover the carbohydrate in your meal.

A commonly used ratio is one unit of rapid-acting insulin per 10g of carbohydrate, or 1:10. This can vary from person to person, and your ratio might end up being 1:15, 2:10, or something else. So, if your ratio was 1:15, eating 45g of carbohydrate with a meal would require you to inject three units of insulin.

Advanced Carbohydrate Counting

For people who have mastered basic carbohydrate counting and wish to move on to a more advanced carbohydrate counting level (e.g., if they are planning to use an insulin pump or a basal-bolus insulin regimen), the following skills are recommended:

- Understanding of target blood glucose levels
- Ability to apply all aspects of basic carbohydrate counting
- Understanding of the action of insulin and the basal-bolus insulin concept
- Ability to carry out pattern management
- Willingness and ability to keep adequate records.

Additional helpful skills include knowing how to calculate a bolus insulin dose using insulin-to-carbohydrate ratios, how to calculate an insulin sensitivity factor for use in the correction or supplementation of insulin doses when glucose levels are too high or too low before meals, and how to make adjustments for special situations.5

Various approaches and methods exist for determining insulin-to-carbohydrate ratios. A general guideline, at least for patients with type 1 diabetes, is that most people need about half of their total daily dose of insulin for basal (background) insulin and half for bolus doses to cover meals. In type 2 diabetes, the basal and bolus needs can vary substantially from person to person. Bolus insulin doses can be calculated from the insulin-to-carbohydrate ratio based on the total grams of carbohydrate or the total number of 15-g carbohydrate servings to be consumed.

How many carbs should I eat?

There's no "one size fits all" answer—everyone is different because everyone's body is different. The amount you can eat and stay in your target blood sugar range depends on your age, weight, activity level, and other factors.

On average, people with diabetes should aim to get about half of their calories from carbs. That means if you normally eat about 1,800 calories a day to maintain a healthy weight, about 800 to 900 calories can come from carbs. At 4 calories per gram, that's 200–225 carb grams a day. Try to eat about the same amount of carbs at each meal to keep your blood sugar levels steady throughout the day (not necessary if you use an insulin pump or give yourself multiple daily injections—you'll take a fast-acting or short-acting insulin at mealtimes to match the amount of carbs you eat).

If you eat packaged foods, a convenient way to figure out how much carbohydrate is in your food is to use the "Nutrition Facts Label." The "Nutrition Facts Label" is found on the outside of the container.

To count carbohydrates, look at three things:

- Serving Size
- Number of Servings Per Container
- Grams of Total Carbohydrate per serving

The total carbohydrate tells how many grams of carbohydrate are in one serving. Be careful when reading the label. There can be more than one serving in the package, so if you eat more than one serving, you will need to multiply the grams of carbohydrate accordingly.

Choose foods with more fiber, vitamins, and minerals.

Choose foods with lower calories, saturated fat, sodium, and added sugars. Avoid trans fat.

Serving Size

A serving size is a standard measurement based on the amount of food people typically have at one time. The size of the serving determines the amounts listed on the label. It helps you figure how many calories and nutrients are in your food on your plate.

Pay attention to that serving size, including the number of servings in the package, and compare it to how much you're actually eating. Don't confuse portion size with serving size. A portion is what you choose to eat -- and there are no standard measures for this.

For example, if a slice of bread is a serving size and you eat a sandwich with two slices of bread, you've had two servings of bread in your one portion, so you'll have to double all the nutritional numbers like calories and carbs. If a package has four servings and you eat the whole thing (like a bag of crunchy snacks), you get 4 times the calories, fat, and everything else listed on the label.

Calories and Calories From Fat

Calories measure energy, so this number tells you how much energy you get from one serving. (Remember, you'll need to adjust this if your portion is different from the serving size on the label.)

his part of the label also tells you how much of that energy comes from the fat in a serving.

Nutrients

"% Daily Value" shows how much a serving of that food gives you for each key nutrient listed. These daily goals are set by the government, based on current nutrition recommendations. The percentages are based on a 2,000 calorie/day diet, which would be right for an average- or large-size man who gets little exercise. Women or seniors with diabetes, or people trying to lose weight, need fewer calories.

Put sugar-free products in their place

Sugar-free doesn't mean carbohydrate-free. Sugar-free foods may play a role in your diabetes diet, but remember that it's equally important to consider carbohydrates as well. A sugar-free label means that one serving has less than 0.5 grams of sugar.

When you're choosing between standard products and their sugar-free counterparts, compare the food labels. If the sugar-free product has noticeably fewer carbohydrates, the sugar-free product might be the better choice. But if there's little difference in carbohydrate grams between the two foods, let taste — or price — be your guide.

No sugar added, but not necessarily no carbohydrates. The same caveat applies to products sporting a "no sugar added" label. These foods don't contain high-sugar ingredients, and no sugar is added during processing or packaging, but they may still be high in carbohydrates.

Sugar alcohols contain carbohydrates and calories, too. Likewise, products that contain sugar alcohols — such as sorbitol, xylitol and mannitol — aren't necessarily low in carbohydrates or calories.

Beware of fat-free products

Per gram, fat has more than twice the calories of carbohydrates or protein. If you're trying to lose weight, fat-free foods might sound like just the ticket. But don't be fooled by "fat-free" food labels.

Fat-free can still have carbohydrates. Fat-free foods can have more carbohydrates and contain nearly as many calories as the standard version of the same food. The lesson? You guessed it. Compare food labels for fat-free and standard products carefully before you make a decision.

And remember that the amount of total fat listed on a food label doesn't tell the whole story. Look for a breakdown of types of fat.

Choose healthier fats. Although still high in calories, monounsaturated and polyunsaturated fats are better choices, as they can help lower your cholesterol and protect your heart.

Limit unhealthy fats. Saturated and trans fats raise your cholesterol and increase your risk of heart disease.

Know what counts as a free food

Just as food labels can help you avoid certain foods, food labels can also serve as your guide to free foods. A free food is one with:

- Fewer than 20 calories a serving
- Less than 5 grams of carbohydrates a serving.

What physical activities should I do if I have diabetes?

Most kinds of physical activity can help you take care of your diabetes. Certain activities may be unsafe for some people, such as those with low vision or nerve damage to their feet. Ask your health care team what physical activities are safe for you. Many people choose walking with friends or family members for their activity.

Doing different types of physical activity each week will give you the most health benefits. Mixing it up also helps reduce boredom and lower your chance of getting hurt. Try these options for physical activity.

Add extra activity to your daily routine

If you have been inactive or you are trying a new activity, start slowly, with 5 to 10 minutes a day. Then add a little more time each week. Increase daily activity by spending less time in front of a TV or other screen. Try these simple ways to add physical activities in your life each day:

Walk around while you talk on the phone or during TV commercials.

Do chores, such as work in the garden, rake leaves, clean the house, or wash the car.

Park at the far end of the shopping center parking lot and walk to the store.

Take the stairs instead of the elevator.

Make your family outings active, such as a family bike ride or a walk in a park.

If you are sitting for a long time, such as working at a desk or watching TV, do some light activity for 3 minutes or more every half hour. Light activities include

- leg lifts or extensions
- overhead arm stretches
- desk chair swivels
- torso twists
- side lunges
- walking in place
- Do aerobic exercise

Aerobic exercise is activity that makes your heart beat faster and makes you breathe harder. You should aim for doing aerobic exercise for 30 minutes a day most days of the week. You do not have to do all the activity at one time. You can split up these

minutes into a few times throughout the
day.

To get the most out of your activity,
exercise at a moderate to vigorous level. Try

- walking briskly or hiking
- climbing stairs
- swimming or a water-aerobics class
- dancing
- riding a bicycle or a stationary bicycle
- taking an exercise class
- playing basketball, tennis, or other
  sports
- Talk with your health care team about
  how to warm up and cool down
  before and after you exercise.

Do strength training to build muscle

Strength training is a light or moderate physical activity that builds muscle and helps keep your bones healthy. Strength training is important for both men and women. When you have more muscle and less body fat, you'll burn more calories. Burning more calories can help you lose and keep off extra weight.

You can do strength training with hand weights, elastic bands, or weight machines. Try to do strength training two to three times a week. Start with a light weight. Slowly increase the size of your weights as your muscles become stronger.

Do stretching exercises

Stretching exercises are light or moderate physical activity. When you stretch, you increase your flexibility, lower your stress, and help prevent sore muscles.

You can choose from many types of stretching exercises. Yoga is a type of stretching that focuses on your breathing and helps you relax. Even if you have problems moving or balancing, certain types of yoga can help. For instance, chair yoga has stretches you can do when sitting in a chair or holding onto a chair while standing. Your health care team can suggest whether yoga is right for you.

How Your Body Handles Sugar Alcohol Carbs

Sugar alcohols are processed similarly to fiber, with a few important differences.

Many sugar alcohols are only partially absorbed in the small intestine, and there is a lot of variation among different types.

Researchers report the small intestine absorbs 2–90% of sugar alcohols. However, some are only briefly absorbed into the bloodstream and then excreted in urine

In addition, these sugar alcohols can have varying effects on blood sugar and insulin levels, although all are considerably lower than sugar.

Here is a list of the glycemic and insulin indexes for the most common sugar alcohols. By comparison, glucose's glycemic and insulin index are both 100

- Erythritol: Glycemic index 0, insulin index 2
- Isomalt: Glycemic index 9, insulin index 6

- Maltitol: Glycemic index 35, insulin index 27
- Sorbitol: Glycemic index 9, insulin index 11

Xylitol: Glycemic index 13, insulin index 11

Maltitol is the most commonly used sugar alcohol in processed foods, including low-carb protein bars and sugar-free candy.

It's partially absorbed in the small intestine, and the remainder is fermented by bacteria in the colon. It's also been found to contribute about 3–3.5 calories per gram, compared with 4 calories per gram for sugar

Anecdotally, maltitol has been reported to increase blood sugar levels in people with diabetes and prediabetes.

In terms of net carbs, erythritol seems to be the best choice all around.

About 90% of it is absorbed in the small intestine and then excreted in the urine. The remaining 10% is fermented to SCFAs in the colon, making it essentially carb-free, calorie-free and unlikely to cause digestive troubles

Studies have shown that other sugar alcohols are also partially absorbed and may raise blood sugar, although to a lesser extent than maltitol. However, they seem to cause significant bloating, gas and loose stools in many people

Importantly, the controlled studies on sugar alcohols involved fewer than 10 people, and blood sugar levels weren't always tested.

Overall, sugar alcohols don't seem to have a major effect on blood sugar and insulin levels, but individual responses may vary, especially among those with diabetes or prediabetes.

Insulin To Carbohydrate Ratio(ICR)

Your insulin-to-carb ratio is a number that tells you how much rapid-acting insulin you need to cover a specific amount of carbohydrate. It's what allows you to accurately dose insulin for meals or to correct high blood sugars.

Counting grams of carbohydrate (or carbohydrate "choices") and using an insulin-to-carbohydrate ratio allows a person to give himself just enough insulin to cover the carbohydrate he plans to eat. This means he doesn't have to eat the exact same amount of carbohydrate for a given meal each day. Knowing how to count carbohydrate and use an insulin-to-carbohydrate ratio is valuable for tightly managing blood glucose levels, and it is essential for using an insulin pump effectively

This sample menu has about 1,800 calories and 200 grams of carbs:

Breakfast

½ cup rolled oats (28g)

1 cup low-fat milk (13g)

2/3 medium banana (20g)

¼ cup chopped walnuts (4g)

Total carbs: 65 grams

Lunch

2 slices whole wheat bread (24g)

4 oz. low-sodium turkey meat (1g)

1 slice low-fat Swiss cheese (1g)

½ large tomato (3g)

1 TBS yellow mustard (1g)

¼ cup shredded lettuce (0g)

8 baby carrots (7g)

6 oz. plain fat-free Greek yogurt (7g)

¾ cup blueberries (15g)

Total carbs: 59 grams

Dinner

6 ounces baked chicken breast (0g)

1 cup brown rice (45g)

1 cup steamed broccoli (12g)

2 TBS margarine (0g)

Total carbs: 57 grams

Snack

1 low-fat string cheese stick (1g)

2 tangerines (18g)

Total carbs: 19 gram

If the timing of your insulin for the meal is off, but your carb count and carb ratio is right, you might see your blood sugar go slightly out of range but it should be back in range within 90 minutes (which is the average time insulin peaks.)

It's also important to note that you should subtract the fiber content in your meal from your total carb count before calculating your insulin dose because fiber doesn't break down completely in your digestive system and therefore does not raise blood sugar levels. Dosing for fiber could lead to a low blood sugar.

How to calculate your carb ratio(s)

To use an insulin-to-carb ratio, you need to:

Plan ahead and eat all of your meal.

Take your rapid-acting insulin 15 minutes before you eat.

The only time it is okay to take the rapid-acting insulin after eating is for very young children who may not eat everything. If a child is taking their insulin after they eat, they must take it as soon as they finish eating, within 30 minutes of their first bite of food.

- Taking insulin after eating will always result in a high blood sugar a few hours later.
- Taking insulin before eating and then not eating all of the planned carbohydrate will result in a low blood sugar when the rapid-acting insulin peaks.

- If you will be using an insulin-to-carb ratio to calculate rapid-acting insulin doses, you will need to be accurate at counting carbohydrate and doing math to calculate your dose.
- Focus on one meal at a time (breakfast for example). Try to enjoy the meal at roughly the same time each day and eat the same foods and quantities for the data collection period (this is why breakfast is a good place to start as its easier to eat the same thing for breakfast each day)
- Make sure your carb count is correct and stick with the same carb ratio for the data collection period
- Try not to do anything that impacts your blood sugar significantly right before or after the meal (like going for a run)

- Be on top of your blood sugar measurements or Continuous Glucose Monitor (CGM)
- Measure your blood sugar before the meal
- Measure your blood sugar after the meal (90-120 minutes after your injection)
- After 3-5 days, you should have enough data to start assessing whether your carb ratio for this time of day is accurate.

When you or your doctor does the analysis, you'll focus on whether your blood sugar was in your desired range before the meal and whether your blood sugar came back into your desired range within 90-120 minutes of your insulin injection.

Insulin-to-Carb Ratios: How to Calculate Insulin Doses

Do you live with insulin-dependent diabetes, count your carbs accurately, but still struggle with postprandial (after meal) high or low blood sugars?

If so, your "insulin-to-carb ratio" may need adjustment.

Your insulin-to-carb ratio is a number that tells you how much rapid-acting insulin you need to cover a specific amount of carbohydrate. It's what allows you to accurately dose insulin for meals or to correct high blood sugars.

In this post, I will cover what your insulin-to-carb ratio is, how to find yours, factors that can influence it, and the available tools and mobile apps that can help you find and keep track of your ratios.

If your doctor is the one changing your insulin-to-carb ratios, a lot of the information we'll discuss in this post will be relevant to bring to your doctor so that he or she can make informed changes to your diabetes management.

What is an insulin-to-carb ratio and why does it matter?

Your insulin-to-carb ratio (also just called a "carb ratio" or "carb factor") indicates how many grams of carbs one unit of rapid-acting insulin covers to ensure that your blood sugars stay in your desired range.

Your carb ratio is often initially set by your doctor when you are diagnosed but should be updated regularly (if needed). A carb ratio of 1:10 means that that 1 unit of rapid-acting insulin will cover 10 grams of carbs. A higher ratio indicates that you need less insulin to cover your carbs.

Let me give you an example:

If my carb ratio is 1:10 and I'm eating 30 grams of carbs, I'll need 3 units of rapid-acting insulin to cover the meal (30 divided by 10), however, if my carb ratio is 1:15 I'll only need 2 units of rapid-acting insulin (30 divided by 15)

That a higher carb ratio means less insulin can take a little time to wrap your head around but it's an important fact when you start adjusting your carb ratio(s).

If you time the peak of your insulin with your meal, an accurate carb count combined with an accurate carb ratio will mean that your blood sugar should stay within your desired range and below 180 mg/dl (10 mmol/L).

If the timing of your insulin for the meal is off, but your carb count and carb ratio is right, you might see your blood sugar go slightly out of range but it should be back in range within 90 minutes (which is the average time insulin peaks.)

It's also important to note that you should subtract the fiber content in your meal from your total carb count before calculating your insulin dose because fiber doesn't break down completely in your digestive system and therefore does not raise blood sugar levels. Dosing for fiber could lead to a low blood sugar.

How to calculate your carb ratio(s)

If you suspect that your carb ratio is off (often running high or low after meals could be a good indicator of that), it's time to collect data in the form of blood sugar readings and do some analysis.

If you want good results you need good data, and you're the only one who can collect it. As with most other things related to diabetes, it requires work but it's worth it.

following the 4 steps below for 3-5 days minimum to collect data for you or your doctor to assess whether your carb ratio is correct. If you and/or your doctor don't see any trends after 3-5 days, you'll have to collect more blood sugar data.

Focus on one meal at a time (breakfast for example). Try to enjoy the meal at roughly the same time each day and eat the same foods and quantities for the data collection period (this is why breakfast is a good place to start as its easier to eat the same thing for breakfast each day)

Make sure your carb count is correct and stick with the same carb ratio for the data collection period

Try not to do anything that impacts your blood sugar significantly right before or after the meal (like going for a run)

Be on top of your blood sugar measurements or Continuous Glucose Monitor (CGM)

Measure your blood sugar before the meal

Measure your blood sugar after the meal (90-120 minutes after your injection)

After 3-5 days, you should have enough data to start assessing whether your carb ratio for this time of day is accurate.

When you or your doctor does the analysis, you'll focus on whether your blood sugar was in your desired range before the meal and whether your blood sugar came back into your desired range within 90-120 minutes of your insulin injection.

Let's look at 2 different scenarios, assuming a meal of 30 carbs (that's counted as accurately as possible) and a starting carb ratio of 1:10.

Blood sugar in-range before the meal, but high 90-120 minutes after

If your blood sugar is not back in range or coming down quickly 90-120 minutes after your meal, your carb ratio is too high. You can consider trying to experiment with ratios below 1:10, maybe 1:9 or 1:8 is the right ratio for you.

Blood sugar in-range before the meal, but low 90-120 minutes after

If your blood sugar is lower than your target range 90-120 minutes after your meal, your carb ratio is too low. You can consider trying to experiment with ratios higher than 1:10, maybe you need to go to 1:11 or 1:12. As mentioned, I usually do small incremental changes.

You also need to consider if your timing for when you take your insulin is off. If you have a low blood sugar within 30-60 minutes of your injection, your food might not have been sufficiently digested yet and will hit your bloodstream later. You can assess this by measuring your blood sugar frequently and experiment with taking your insulin a little later.

Note: The carb ratios listed here are just examples. You can have ratios much higher or lower than 1:10.

When deciding whether to round up or down, think about:

Rounding up if your blood sugar is high

Rounding down if your blood sugar is low

What you will be doing in the next few hours, such as being active or sitting around

This can be confusing at first, but doing the math can help you understand this better.

Changing the insulin-to-carb ratio

You will have to do some math to figure out how to change your ratio. The diabetes nurses will teach you how to do this. It will not be perfect at first. It will take some time.

Things to remember in order to change insulin doses:

If the pattern happens at the blood sugar check before breakfast, change the long-acting insulin dose by 10 percent.

If the pattern happens at the blood sugar check before lunch, change the breakfast rapid-acting insulin dose by 10 percent.

If the pattern happens at the blood sugar check 2 to 3 hours after lunch, change the lunch rapid-acting insulin dose by 10 percent.

If the pattern happens at the blood sugar check 2 to 3 hours after supper (before the bedtime snack), change the supper rapid-acting insulin dose by 10 percent.

If your blood sugar is above 180 two to three hours after a meal, ask yourself what caused this.

Common reasons for high blood sugar 2 to 3 hours after eating are:

Not taking insulin at least 15 minutes before eating

Eating too much carbohydrate or too much quick-acting carbohydrate

Not taking enough insulin to cover the carbohydrate

Not eating protein or fat in your meal

Eating a very high fat meal

Things that influence your carb ratios

Our bodies change over time and so does our eating and exercise patterns. And as your body and daily routine changes, you might find that your carb ratio(s) needs to be adjusted.

Here are things that can influence your carb ratios:

Time of day

You might have noticed that I write "carb ratio(s)" because most people have more than one carb ratio. For example, many are more insulin resistant in the morning so they might need a lower carb ratio for breakfast than they do for lunch or dinner.

In theory, you can have as many carb ratios as you like, but most diabetes devices (pumps, apps, smartpens) have a limited number..

Time of month (for women)

The fluctuating hormone levels of your menstruation cycle can have a significant impact on your blood sugars and your insulin needs. This can mean that you need different carb ratios (and most likely basal insulin) for periods where you're extra insulin resistant due to hormonal changes.

I'm one of those women who see large differences in my insulin needs throughout my cycle. I need significantly less insulin the day(s) right before my period and always need to increase my carb ratios.

Type of meal: the impact of protein & fat

Carbs might be what's converted into glucose in the bloodstream the fastest, but it's not the only macronutrient that can impact your blood sugar.

If you eat large amounts of protein, you'll most likely need to inject insulin to not see an increase in your blood sugar.

If you add large amounts of fat to your meal, you'll most likely see a delayed release of the glucose into your bloodstream, which for many people means that they need to take two insulin doses rather than just one (one with the meal and one some time later).

Bodyweight

If your bodyweight changes significantly, you'll most likely see that your insulin needs change as well.

If your bodyfat percentage increases significantly, you might experience that you need more insulin to cover your meals. If you gain a significant amount of muscle mass, on the other hand, you might see that you need less insulin to cover your meals.

Tools to help you find and remember your carb ratios

Using carb ratios is pretty straight forward if you use an insulin pump to manage your diabetes. Most pumps have a build-in bolus calculator (calculates your suggested dose) and your medical team should have set it up for you and trained you on how to use it. If that's the case, you just need to focus on whether your ratios are accurate.

If you manage your diabetes with manual injections, you need to look elsewhere for a "carb calculator" or memorize or write down your ratio(s). The benefit of a good calculator is that it can keep track of active insulin (insulin lasts 3-5 hours in the body) and can help keep track of your injections and ratio(s).

Mobile apps: There are no FDA approved standalone apps that are approved for dosing recommendations in the United States, but I have used RapidCalc (not-FDA approved) and found it to be accurate and easy to use.

Outside of the United States, good options are the Hedia and MySugr apps.

Smart insulin pens: Companion Medical's InPen is a smartpen available in the US only. It has all the functionalities of a pump, except for actually pumping, so it automatically keeps track of active insulin and has a bolus calculator. It sends the data directly to your phone via Bluetooth.

Novo Nordisk has announced that they expect to launch their smartpens in 2020.

Smart meters: Some blood glucose meters also have bolus calculator functionalities or have an app that links with the meter.

Challenges and Advantages of Carbohydrate Counting

carbohydrate counting offers several strong advantages. It is single-nutrient focused, provides a more precise method of matching food and mealtime insulin, allows flexibility of food choices, creates potential for improved blood glucose control, and is empowering to patients. Understanding the need to adjust insulin for larger or smaller meals, knowing one's own pre- and postmeal blood glucose targets, using pattern management skills, and calculating bolus and basal insulin doses can all help people with diabetes be successful in using this meal planning system.

Nutrition labels on packaged foods make it easy to count carbs.

Keeping a target carb number in mind is a tangible measure of how much to eat

Challenges

In type 1 diabetes, which affects about 3 million Americans, the pancreas doesn't produce sufficient amounts of the hormone insulin, which helps ferry sugar from the blood into cells. So people with the disease are quickly overwhelmed when the sugar in their food hits the bloodstream.

To avoid the dangerous blood sugar surge, diabetics inject insulin before a meal -- usually based on how many carbohydrates they will be downing.

Keeping track of carbohydrates alone does not necessarily equate to a healthy diet

It may be easier to rely on packaged foods with nutrition labels than whole foods like fruits and vegetables, which don't have carbs listed on them

Not all foods contain carbohydrates, but still may be high in calories and fat, such as steak or bacon—this can become hard to track if you're only counting carbs.

carb counting can be a healthy way to manage blood sugar and make it easy to visualize and keep track of your intake, but that the quality of the carbs you're eating does matter. For best results, focus your carb choices on high-quality, less processed foods such as whole grains, fresh or frozen fruit, and vegetables.

Calculating net carbs is one way to do this. The term "net carbs" simply refers to carbs that are absorbed by the body.

To calculate the net carbs in whole foods, subtract the fiber from the total number of carbs. To calculate the net carbs in processed foods, subtract the fiber and a portion of the sugar alcohols.

Nevertheless, remember that the "net carbs" listed on food labels can be misleading, and individual responses may also vary.

If you find that counting net carbs leads to higher-than-expected blood sugar levels or other issues, you may prefer to count total carbs instead. The key is to eat the number of carbs that allows you to achieve your health goals, no matter how you count them